A COMPREHENSIVE ANTI PARKINSON'S DIET COOKBOOK: EAT YOUR WAY TO WELLNESS

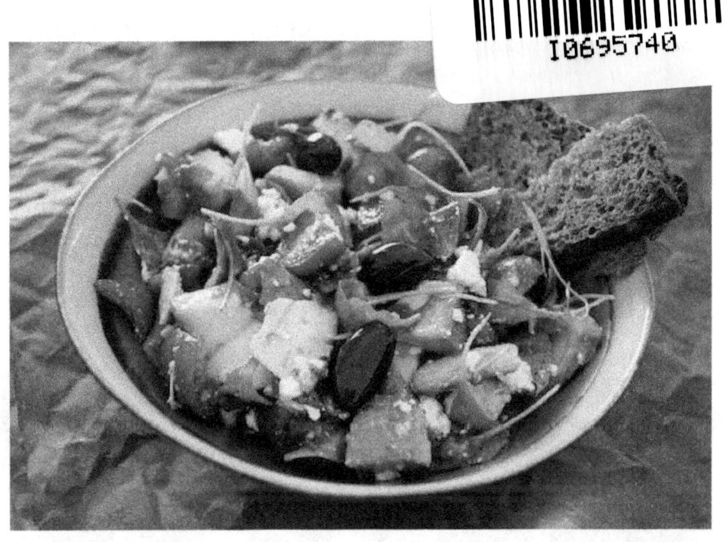

Dr. Becca Smith

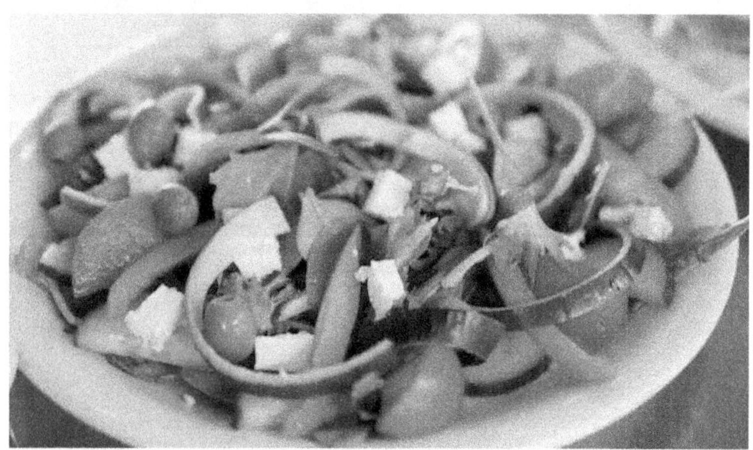

TABLE OF CONTENT

INTRODUCTION

In a quaint village nestled between rolling hills, lived a brilliant young woman named Eliza. She had always been captivated by the mysteries of the human body and had dedicated her life to unraveling them. Her focus was on Parkinson's disease, a formidable foe that affected the lives of many in her community.

Eliza tirelessly researched the intricate connections between diet and neurodegenerative diseases. She spent countless hours poring over medical journals and studies, seeking the missing link that could potentially lead to a breakthrough. Her dedication led her to discover a compelling correlation between certain nutrients and the progression of Parkinson's.

Armed with her newfound insights, Eliza embarked on a mission to develop a specialized diet tailored to counteract the effects of the disease.

She combined foods rich in antioxidants, essential fatty acids, and nutrients known to support brain health. Eliza's diet plan was met with skepticism initially, but she remained steadfast in her conviction.

As time passed, word of Eliza's remarkable research spread far and wide. People from various corners of the world sought her guidance and embraced her dietary recommendations. One particular patient, Michael, had been battling severe Parkinson's symptoms for years. Traditional treatments had offered minimal relief, leaving him desperate for a solution.

With Eliza's guidance, Michael wholeheartedly adopted the specialized diet. He incorporated colorful fruits and vegetables, lean proteins, and omega-3 fatty acids into his meals. Gradually, he noticed subtle changes—a tremor that had plagued him for years began to ease, his mobility improved, and his overall sense of well-being was on the rise.

Months turned into years, and the change in Michael's condition was nothing short of astonishing. His once debilitating symptoms had significantly receded, allowing him to engage in activities he had long given up on. Eliza's breakthrough dietary approach had not only halted the progression of his Parkinson's disease but had actually reversed some of its effects.

News of Michael's remarkable recovery spread like wildfire, catapulting Eliza into the spotlight. Medical professionals and researchers marveled at her groundbreaking work, acknowledging the undeniable impact of her dietary approach on Parkinson's patients.

Eliza's village transformed into a hub of hope and healing, where individuals from all walks of life gathered to learn and embrace the power of nutrition.

Eliza's journey was a testament to the remarkable influence one person's dedication and determination could have on the world.

Through her relentless pursuit of knowledge, she had shattered the boundaries of conventional medicine and opened new avenues of treatment for Parkinson's disease. Her legacy endured as a beacon of inspiration, reminding us all that sometimes, the cure we seek may lie within the simplest of solutions.

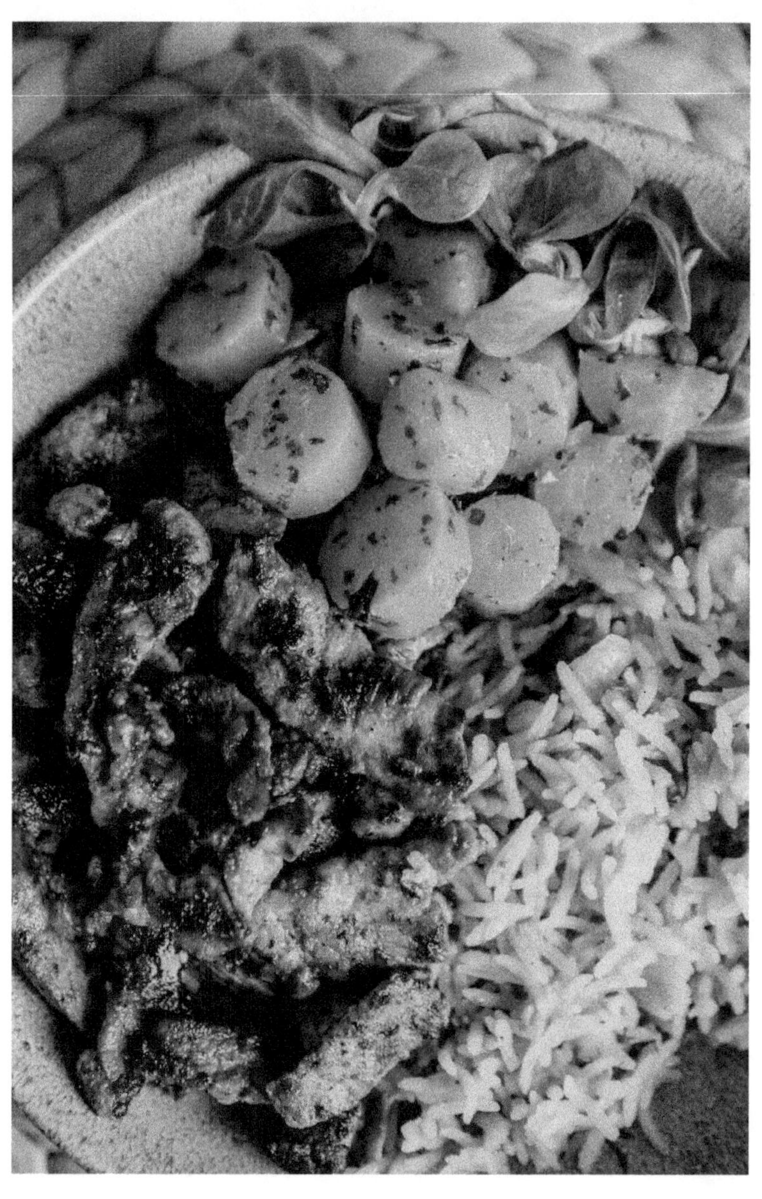

CHAPTER ONE

Types, Causes and Symptoms of Anti Parkinson Disease

Parkinson's disease is a complex neurodegenerative disorder that affects millions of people worldwide. It's characterized by a range of motor and non-motor symptoms that can significantly impact a person's quality of life. While there isn't a definitive cure for Parkinson's disease, advancements in research and treatment options have improved the management of its symptoms.

Parkinson's disease is not an "anti" disease, but rather a condition on its own. However, it seems you might be referring to treatments that aim to counteract Parkinson's symptoms, which we can explore. Let's delve into the different types, causes, and symptoms of Parkinson's disease:

Types of Parkinson's Disease

1. Idiopathic Parkinson's Disease: This is the most common form of Parkinson's and occurs with no apparent cause.

2. Young-Onset Parkinson's Disease: When symptoms appear before the age of 50, it's termed as young-onset Parkinson's.

3. Secondary Parkinsonism: This refers to similar symptoms caused by underlying conditions or medication side effects.

Causes of Parkinson's Disease

1. Neurodegeneration: The primary cause is the gradual degeneration of dopamine-producing neurons in the substantia nigra region of the brain.

2. Genetics: Some cases have a genetic component, where specific mutations increase the risk of developing Parkinson's.

3. Environmental Factors: Exposure to certain toxins and pesticides has been linked to an increased risk of Parkinson's disease.

4. Alpha-Synuclein Accumulation: The buildup of misfolded alpha-synuclein protein in brain cells contributes to Parkinson's pathology.

Symptoms of Parkinson's Disease

1. Motor Symptoms:

- Tremors: Involuntary shaking, often starting in the hands.
- Bradykinesia: Slowness of movement, making simple tasks challenging.
- Rigidity: Stiffness and resistance in muscles, leading to decreased flexibility.
- Postural Instability: Difficulty maintaining balance, increasing the risk of falls.

2. Non-Motor Symptoms

- Depression: Feelings of sadness, apathy, and lack of interest.
- Sleep Disturbances: Insomnia, restless legs, and rapid eye movement (REM) sleep behavior disorder.
- Cognitive Changes: Memory problems, slowed thinking, and difficulty multitasking.
- Autonomic Dysfunction: Issues with blood pressure regulation, digestion, and urinary function.
- Speech and Swallowing Issues: Soft speech, slurring, and difficulty swallowing.

Anti Parkinson Diet with Benefits

Parkinson's disease is a progressive neurodegenerative disorder that impacts millions of lives worldwide. While there is no cure, emerging research suggests that adopting a carefully curated diet can help manage its symptoms and potentially slow down its progression. An anti-Parkinson's diet, rich in specific nutrients, antioxidants, and anti-inflammatory compounds, has shown promise in enhancing the quality of life for those living with this condition.

Understanding the Anti-Parkinson's Diet:

An anti-Parkinson's diet focuses on providing essential nutrients that support brain health and minimize oxidative stress, inflammation, and the loss of dopamine-producing neurons. While not a standalone treatment, when combined with medical therapies and other interventions, this diet can contribute significantly to symptom management.

Key Components of an Anti-Parkinson's Diet

1. Antioxidant-Rich Foods

Incorporate a rainbow of fruits and vegetables such as berries, spinach, kale, broccoli, and bell peppers. These foods are packed with antioxidants that combat free radicals, which contribute to neurodegeneration.

2. Omega-3 Fatty Acids

Include sources of omega-3 fatty acids, like fatty fish (salmon, mackerel, sardines), flaxseeds, and walnuts. Omega-3s possess anti-inflammatory properties and support brain function.

3. Lean Proteins

Opt for lean protein sources like poultry, fish, beans, lentils, and tofu. Protein is essential for muscle maintenance and overall health, but a balance is crucial to prevent excessive protein intake, which may interfere with levodopa absorption.

4. Whole Grains:

Choose whole grains such as brown rice, quinoa, whole wheat, and oats. These provide sustained energy and fiber that supports gut health and regulates blood sugar levels.

5. Vitamin D:

Exposure to sunlight and vitamin D-rich foods like fortified dairy, eggs, and fatty fish can contribute to bone health and may play a role in managing Parkinson's symptoms.

6. B Vitamins:

Consume foods rich in B vitamins, particularly B6, B12, and folate. These vitamins support nerve function and may aid in reducing homocysteine levels associated with neurodegeneration.

7. Curcumin and Turmeric:

Turmeric, with its active compound curcumin, has shown anti-inflammatory and antioxidant effects. Incorporate it into your cooking or consider curcumin supplements after consulting a healthcare professional.

Benefits of an Anti-Parkinson's Diet:

1. Neuroprotective Effects:

Antioxidants and anti-inflammatory compounds in the diet may help protect brain cells from damage and oxidative stress, potentially slowing down the progression of the disease.

2. Improved Gut Health:

Emerging research suggests a link between gut health and Parkinson's.

A diet rich in fiber and probiotics (found in yogurt, kefir, and fermented foods) can support a healthy gut microbiome, which may positively impact Parkinson's symptoms.

3. Enhanced Mood and Mental Health:

Omega-3 fatty acids and nutrient-rich foods can promote better mental health, potentially reducing symptoms of depression and anxiety that often accompany Parkinson's disease.

4. Stabilized Energy Levels:

A balanced diet with complex carbohydrates can help regulate blood sugar levels, preventing energy spikes and crashes that can exacerbate motor and non-motor symptoms.

5. Potential Levodopa Enhancement:

Strategic protein intake can improve the effectiveness of levodopa, a common medication used to manage Parkinson's symptoms, by minimizing competition for absorption.

While an anti-Parkinson's diet is not a standalone cure, it plays a vital role in supporting overall well-being and managing symptoms. Consult with a healthcare professional or a registered dietitian before making significant dietary changes.

Remember that every individual's nutritional needs are unique, and a personalized approach can help harness the benefits of an anti-Parkinson's diet, improving the quality of life for those on this journey of resilience and hope.

CHAPTER TWO

A 14-Day Anti Parkinson Disease Diet Meal Plan

Day 1

- Breakfast: Scrambled eggs with spinach and tomatoes, whole-grain toast, and a side of mixed berries.
- Lunch: Grilled chicken salad with mixed greens, bell peppers, cucumber, walnuts, and a light vinaigrette dressing.
- Snack: Greek yogurt with a sprinkle of flaxseeds.
- Dinner: Baked salmon with quinoa, steamed broccoli, and a side salad.

Day 2

- Breakfast: Overnight oats made with rolled oats, almond milk, chia seeds, and topped with sliced banana and a drizzle of honey.
- Lunch: Lentil soup with a side of whole-grain crackers and a side salad.
- Snack: Carrot and celery sticks with hummus.
- Dinner: Stir-fried tofu with mixed vegetables (broccoli, bell peppers, snap peas) and brown rice.

Day 3

- Breakfast: Smoothie with spinach, frozen berries, banana, almond milk, and a tablespoon of ground flaxseeds.
- Lunch: Grilled vegetable wrap with hummus in a whole-grain tortilla.
- Snack: Handful of mixed nuts (walnuts, almonds, cashews).
- Dinner: Baked chicken with sweet potato mash and steamed asparagus.

Day 4

- Breakfast: Scrambled eggs with sautéed mushrooms and whole-grain toast.
- Lunch: Quinoa salad with chickpeas, cherry tomatoes, red onion, feta cheese, and a lemon-tahini dressing.
- Snack: Apple slices with almond butter.
- Dinner: Grilled fish with roasted Brussels sprouts and a side salad.

Day 5

- Breakfast: Greek yogurt parfait with granola, mixed

berries, and a drizzle of honey.

- Lunch: Spinach and kale salad with grilled chicken, strawberries, almonds, and balsamic vinaigrette.

- Snack: Cottage cheese with sliced peaches.

- Dinner: Lentil and vegetable curry served with brown rice.

Day 6

- Breakfast: Whole-grain toast with avocado spread, poached eggs, and a side of orange slices.

- Lunch: Turkey and avocado wrap in a whole-grain tortilla with a side of carrot sticks.

- Snack: Rice cakes with almond butter and banana slices.

- Dinner: Stir-fried shrimp with broccoli, bell peppers, and brown rice.

Day 7

- Breakfast: Chia seed pudding made with almond milk, topped with sliced kiwi and a sprinkle of chopped nuts.

- Lunch: Quinoa and black bean bowl with roasted vegetables and a drizzle of olive oil.
- Snack: Trail mix with dried cranberries, pumpkin seeds, and dark chocolate chips.
- Dinner: Grilled vegetable platter with tofu skewers and a side salad.

Day 8

- Breakfast: Scrambled eggs with spinach and tomatoes, whole-grain toast, and a side of mixed berries.
- Lunch: Grilled chicken salad with mixed greens, bell peppers, cucumber, walnuts, and a light vinaigrette dressing.
- Snack: Greek yogurt with a sprinkle of flaxseeds.
- Dinner: Baked salmon with quinoa, steamed broccoli, and a side salad.

Day 9

- Breakfast: Overnight oats made with rolled oats, almond milk, chia seeds, and topped with sliced banana and a drizzle of honey.

- Lunch: Lentil soup with a side of whole-grain crackers and a side salad.
- Snack: Carrot and celery sticks with hummus.
- Dinner: Stir-fried tofu with mixed vegetables (broccoli, bell peppers, snap peas) and brown rice.

Day 10

- Breakfast: Smoothie with spinach, frozen berries, banana, almond milk, and a tablespoon of ground flaxseeds.
- Lunch: Grilled vegetable wrap with hummus in a whole-grain tortilla.
- Snack: Handful of mixed nuts (walnuts, almonds, cashews).
- Dinner: Baked chicken with sweet potato mash and steamed asparagus.

Day 11

- Breakfast: Scrambled eggs with sautéed mushrooms and whole-grain toast.

- Lunch: Quinoa salad with chickpeas, cherry tomatoes, red onion, feta cheese, and a lemon-tahini dressing.
- Snack: Apple slices with almond butter.
- Dinner: Grilled fish with roasted Brussels sprouts and a side salad.

Day 12

- Breakfast: Greek yogurt parfait with granola, mixed berries, and a drizzle of honey.
- Lunch: Spinach and kale salad with grilled chicken, strawberries, almonds, and balsamic vinaigrette.
- Snack: Cottage cheese with sliced peaches.
- Dinner: Lentil and vegetable curry served with brown rice.

Day 13:

- Breakfast: Whole-grain toast with avocado spread, poached eggs, and a side of orange slices.
- Lunch: Turkey and avocado wrap in a whole-grain tortilla with a side of carrot sticks.
- Snack: Rice cakes with almond butter and banana slices.
- Dinner: Stir-fried shrimp with broccoli, bell peppers, and brown rice.

Day 14

- Breakfast: Chia seed pudding made with almond milk, topped with sliced kiwi and a sprinkle of chopped nuts.

- Lunch: Quinoa and black bean bowl with roasted vegetables and a drizzle of olive oil.
- Snack: Trail mix with dried cranberries, pumpkin seeds, and dark chocolate chips.
- Dinner: Grilled vegetable platter with tofu skewers and a side salad.

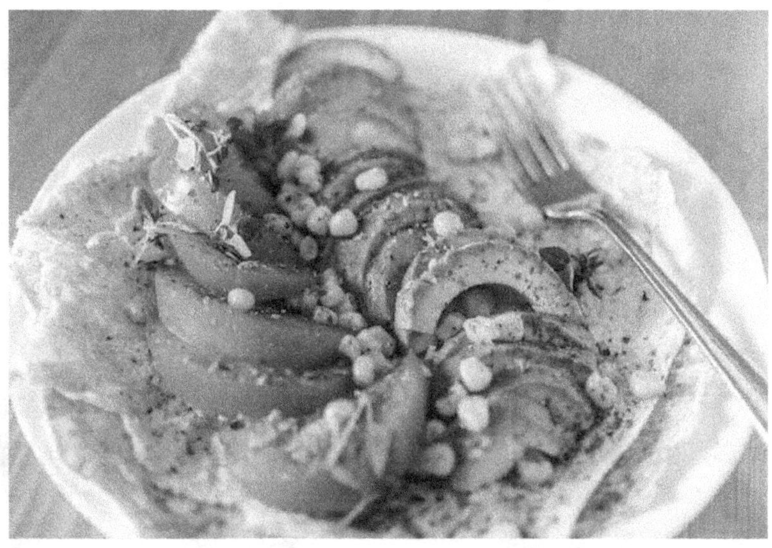

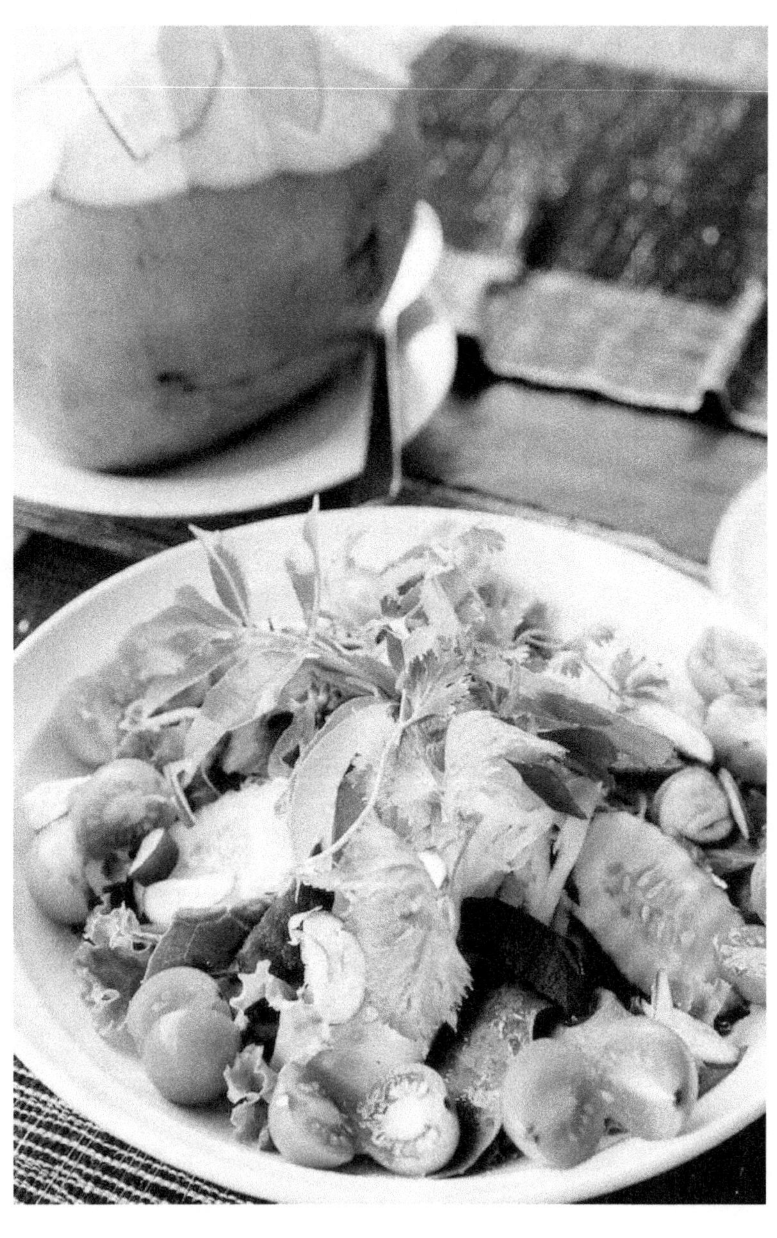

CHAPTER THREE

Anti-Parkinson's Disease Diet Breakfast Recipes

1. Berry Spinach Power Smoothie

Ingredients:

- 1 cup spinach leaves
- 1/2 cup mixed berries (blueberries, strawberries, raspberries)
- 1/2 banana
- 1 tablespoon chia seeds
- 1/2 cup almond milk (or preferred milk)
- 1/4 cup Greek yogurt
- Honey or maple syrup (optional, for sweetness)

Instructions:

1. In a blender, combine spinach, mixed berries, banana, chia seeds, almond milk, and Greek yogurt.
2. Blend until smooth and creamy.
3. Taste and add honey or maple syrup if desired.
4. Pour into a glass and enjoy your antioxidant-packed breakfast.

Cooking Time: 5 minutes

2. Avocado and Egg Breakfast Toast

Ingredients:

- 1 slice whole-grain bread

- 1/2 avocado, sliced

- 1 poached or fried egg

- Salt and pepper to taste

- Red pepper flakes (optional, for a kick)

Instructions:

1. Toast the whole-grain bread.
2. Arrange avocado slices on the toast.
3. Top with a poached or fried egg.
4. Season with salt, pepper, and red pepper flakes.
5. Enjoy this protein-rich breakfast that provides healthy fats and essential nutrients.

Cooking Time: 10 minutes

3. Greek Yogurt Parfait

Ingredients:

- 1/2 cup Greek yogurt

- 1/4 cup granola

- 1/4 cup mixed berries (blueberries, raspberries,

strawberries)

- 1 tablespoon chopped nuts (almonds, walnuts)

Instructions:

1. In a glass or bowl, layer Greek yogurt, granola, mixed berries, and chopped nuts.
2. Repeat the layers.
3. Finish with a sprinkle of nuts on top.
4. Delight in this protein-packed, nutrient-rich breakfast parfait.

    Cooking Time: 5 minutes

4. Overnight Oats with Banana and Almond Butter

Ingredients:

- 1/2 cup rolled oats
- 1/2 cup almond milk
- 1/2 banana, mashed
- 1 tablespoon chia seeds
- 1 tablespoon almond butter

Instructions:

1. In a jar or container, combine rolled oats, almond

milk, mashed banana, and chia seeds.

2. Stir well, cover, and refrigerate overnight.

3. In the morning, give the oats a stir and top with almond butter.

4. Savor these creamy overnight oats that provide fiber and healthy fats.

Cooking Time: Overnight (5 minutes of prep)

5. Whole Grain Pancakes with Mixed Berries

Ingredients:

-   1/2 cup whole wheat flour

-   1/2 cup oat flour

-   1 teaspoon baking powder

-   1 tablespoon ground flaxseeds

-   1 egg

-   1/2 cup almond milk

-   1 tablespoon honey or maple syrup

-   Mixed berries for topping

Instructions:

1. In a bowl, whisk together whole wheat flour, oat flour, baking powder, and ground flaxseeds.

2. In another bowl, beat the egg and mix in almond milk and honey/maple syrup.

3. Combine wet and dry ingredients and stir until just combined.

4. Heat a non-stick pan over medium heat and pour batter to make pancakes.

5. Cook until bubbles form on the surface, then flip and cook until golden brown.

6. Top with mixed berries and enjoy these nutrient-dense pancakes.

Cooking Time: 20 minutes

Anti-Parkinson's Disease Diet Lunch Recipes

1. Grilled Chicken and Quinoa Salad

Ingredients:

- 4 oz grilled chicken breast, sliced

- 1 cup cooked quinoa

- Mixed greens (spinach, kale, arugula)

- Cherry tomatoes, halved

- Cucumber, sliced

- Red onion, thinly sliced

- Balsamic vinaigrette dressing

Instructions:

1. In a bowl, layer mixed greens, cooked quinoa, grilled chicken, cherry tomatoes, cucumber, and red onion.
2. Drizzle with balsamic vinaigrette dressing.
3. Toss gently to combine and enjoy this protein-packed salad.

Cooking Time: 15 minutes (assuming pre-cooked quinoa and grilled chicken)

2. Lentil and Vegetable Stir-Fry

Ingredients:

- 1 cup cooked green lentils

- Mixed vegetables (bell peppers, broccoli, carrots), chopped

- Garlic, minced

- Low-sodium soy sauce

- Sesame oil

- Red pepper flakes (optional, for heat)

- Brown rice or quinoa (optional, for serving)

Instructions:

1. Heat sesame oil in a pan and sauté minced garlic until fragrant.

2. Add chopped mixed vegetables and cook until slightly tender.

3. Add cooked green lentils and a splash of low-sodium soy sauce.

4. Toss everything together and cook for a few more minutes.

5. Serve over brown rice or quinoa if desired.

Cooking Time: 20 minutes

3. Spinach and Chickpea Salad with Tahini Dressing

Ingredients:

- 2 cups baby spinach leaves
- 1 cup canned chickpeas, drained and rinsed
- Red bell pepper, diced
- Red onion, thinly sliced
- Cucumber, chopped
- Feta cheese, crumbled

-   Tahini dressing (tahini, lemon juice, water, salt)

Instructions:

1. In a bowl, combine baby spinach, chickpeas, red bell pepper, red onion, cucumber, and feta cheese.
2. Drizzle with tahini dressing.
3. Toss gently to coat the ingredients and enjoy this nutrient-rich salad.

Cooking Time: 15 minutes

4. Vegetable and Tofu Stir-Fry

Ingredients:

-   4 oz firm tofu, cubed
-   Mixed vegetables (broccoli, snap peas, bell peppers), sliced
-   Ginger, minced
-   Low-sodium stir-fry sauce
-   Brown rice or quinoa (optional, for serving)

Instructions:

1. In a pan, sauté cubed tofu until lightly browned. Set

aside.

2.

3. In the same pan, sauté minced ginger and mixed vegetables until tender.

4. Add the tofu back to the pan and stir in low-sodium stir-fry sauce.

5. Cook for a few more minutes, then serve over brown rice or quinoa if desired.

Cooking Time: 20 minutes

5. Mediterranean Hummus Wrap

Ingredients:

-   Whole-grain tortilla

-   Hummus

-   Grilled chicken or chickpeas (for protein)

-   Cucumber, sliced

-   Tomato, sliced

-   Red onion, thinly sliced

-   Kalamata olives, chopped

-   Feta cheese, crumbled

Instructions:

1. Lay out a whole-grain tortilla.

2. Spread a generous layer of hummus on the tortilla.

3. Add grilled chicken or chickpeas, cucumber, tomato, red onion, kalamata olives, and feta cheese.

4. Roll up the tortilla into a wrap and enjoy this Mediterranean-inspired delight.

Cooking Time: 10 minutes (assuming pre-cooked chicken or chickpeas)

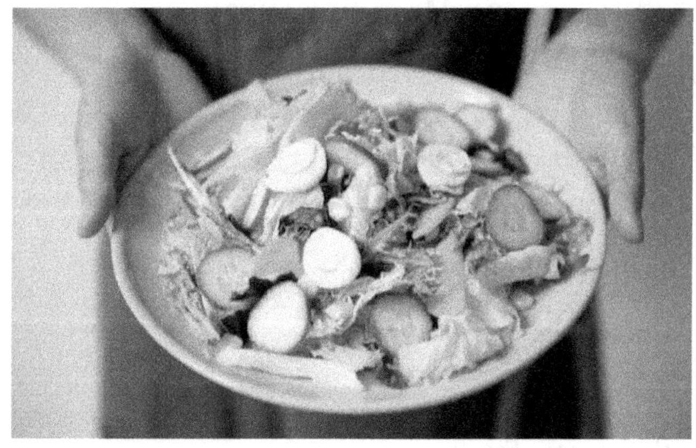

Anti-Parkinson's Disease Diet Dinner Recipes

1. Baked Salmon with Quinoa and Steamed Broccoli

Ingredients:

- 1 salmon fillet
- Lemon juice
- Fresh dill or parsley, chopped
- Salt and pepper
- 1/2 cup cooked quinoa
- Steamed broccoli

Instructions:

1. Preheat the oven to 375°F (190°C).
2. Place the salmon fillet on a baking sheet lined with parchment paper.
3. Drizzle lemon juice over the salmon, sprinkle with chopped dill or parsley, and season with salt and pepper.
4. Bake for about 15-20 minutes, or until the salmon is cooked through.
5. Serve with cooked quinoa and steamed broccoli on the side.

Cooking Time: 25 minutes

2. Veggie-Stuffed Bell Peppers

Ingredients:

- Bell peppers, halved and seeds removed
- Lean ground turkey or tofu crumbles
- Quinoa or brown rice
- Onion, diced
- Garlic, minced
- Mixed vegetables (zucchini, corn, peas)
- Tomato sauce
- Italian seasoning
- Shredded mozzarella cheese (optional)

Instructions:

1. Preheat the oven to 375°F (190°C).
2. In a skillet, cook lean ground turkey or tofu crumbles until browned. Remove from the skillet and set aside.
3. In the same skillet, sauté diced onion, minced garlic, and mixed vegetables until tender.
4. Add cooked quinoa or brown rice, cooked protein, tomato sauce, and Italian seasoning. Mix well.
5. Stuff the halved bell peppers with the mixture and place them in a baking dish.
6. If desired, sprinkle shredded mozzarella cheese on top.
7. Bake for 20-25 minutes, or until the peppers are tender.

Cooking Time: 40 minutes

3. Lentil and Vegetable Curry

Ingredients:

- 1 cup cooked green or brown lentils
- Mixed vegetables (carrots, bell peppers, cauliflower), diced
- Onion, diced
- Garlic, minced
- Curry powder or paste
- Coconut milk
- Fresh cilantro, chopped (for garnish)
- Brown rice or whole-grain naan (optional, for serving)

Instructions:

1. In a large pan, sauté diced onion and minced garlic until fragrant.
2. Add diced mixed vegetables and cook until slightly tender.
3. Stir in curry powder or paste and cook for another minute.
4. Pour in coconut milk and cooked lentils. Simmer until heated through.
5. Serve over brown rice or with whole-grain naan, garnished with chopped cilantro.

Cooking Time: 30 minutes

4. Grilled Vegetable and Chicken Skewers

Ingredients:

- Boneless, skinless chicken breast, cubed
- Assorted vegetables (bell peppers, zucchini, red onion), cut into chunks
- Olive oil
- Lemon juice
- Garlic powder
- Italian seasoning
- Salt and pepper

Instructions:

1. Preheat the grill or grill pan over medium-high heat.
2. Thread chicken and vegetable chunks onto skewers.
3. Drizzle olive oil and lemon juice over the skewers, and sprinkle with garlic powder, Italian seasoning, salt, and pepper.
4. Grill for 10-15 minutes, turning occasionally, until the chicken is cooked through and vegetables are tender.
5. Serve with a side salad or whole-grain bread.

Cooking Time: 20 minutes

5. Quinoa Stuffed Acorn Squash

Ingredients:

- Acorn squash, halved and seeds removed
- 1 cup cooked quinoa

- Ground turkey or plant-based protein (e.g., lentils)
- Onion, diced
- Apple, diced
- Dried cranberries or raisins
- Ground cinnamon
- Nutmeg
- Chopped pecans or walnuts (optional)

Instructions:

1. Preheat the oven to 375°F (190°C).
2. Place the acorn squash halves on a baking sheet.
3. In a skillet, cook ground turkey or plant-based protein until browned. Remove from the skillet and set aside.
4. In the same skillet, sauté diced onion and diced apple until tender.
5. Combine cooked quinoa, cooked protein, sautéed onion and apple, dried cranberries or raisins, ground cinnamon, and nutmeg.
6. Stuff the acorn squash halves with the quinoa mixture.
7. Bake for 30-40 minutes, or until the squash is tender.
8. If desired, sprinkle chopped pecans or walnuts on top before serving.

Cooking Time: 50 minutes

Anti-Parkinson's Disease Diet Dessert Recipes

1. Mixed Berry Parfait

Ingredients:

- Mixed berries (blueberries, strawberries, raspberries)
- Greek yogurt
- Honey or maple syrup
- Chopped nuts (walnuts, almonds)

Instructions:

1. In a glass or bowl, layer mixed berries and Greek yogurt.
2. Drizzle with honey or maple syrup for added sweetness.
3. Sprinkle chopped nuts on top for a crunch.
4. Enjoy this simple and antioxidant-rich dessert.

Preparation Time: 5 minutes

2. Chia Seed Pudding with Mango

Ingredients:

- Chia seeds
- Almond milk or coconut milk
- Vanilla extract
- Fresh mango, diced

Instructions:

1. In a bowl, mix chia seeds, almond milk or coconut milk, and a splash of vanilla extract.
2. Stir well and refrigerate for a few hours or overnight to allow the chia seeds to thicken.
3. Top with diced fresh mango before serving.
4. Savor this creamy and omega-3-rich dessert.

Preparation Time: 5 minutes (plus chilling time)

3. Dark Chocolate-Dipped Strawberries

Ingredients:

-   Fresh strawberries, washed and dried

-   Dark chocolate (70% cocoa or higher)

-   Chopped nuts or shredded coconut (optional, for coating)

Instructions:

1. Melt dark chocolate in a microwave or double boiler.
2. Dip each strawberry into the melted chocolate, coating about half of the berry.
3. Place the dipped strawberries on a parchment-lined tray.
4. If desired, sprinkle chopped nuts or shredded coconut on the chocolate before it sets.
5. Allow the chocolate to harden before enjoying these antioxidant-rich treats.

Preparation Time: 15 minutes

4. Banana-Oat Cookies

Ingredients:

- Ripe bananas, mashed
- Rolled oats
- Cinnamon
- Chopped nuts or dark chocolate chips (optional)

Instructions:

1. Preheat the oven to 350°F (175°C).
2. In a bowl, combine mashed ripe bananas, rolled oats, and a sprinkle of cinnamon.
3. If desired, fold in chopped nuts or dark chocolate chips.
4. Drop spoonful(s) of the mixture onto a baking sheet lined with parchment paper.
5. Bake for about 12-15 minutes, or until the cookies are golden and set.
6. Let them cool before indulging in these naturally sweetened cookies.

Preparation Time: 20 minutes

5. Coconut-Berry Frozen Yogurt Bites

Ingredients:

- Greek yogurt

- Shredded coconut
- Mixed berries (blueberries, raspberries)
- Honey or maple syrup (optional)

Instructions:

1. In a bowl, mix Greek yogurt with shredded coconut.
2. Spoon the mixture into mini muffin cups or silicone molds, filling them halfway.
3. Add a few mixed berries on top of each yogurt-filled cup.
4. Drizzle honey or maple syrup over the berries if desired.
5. Freeze until firm, then pop out the yogurt bites and enjoy.

Preparation Time: 10 minutes (plus freezing time)

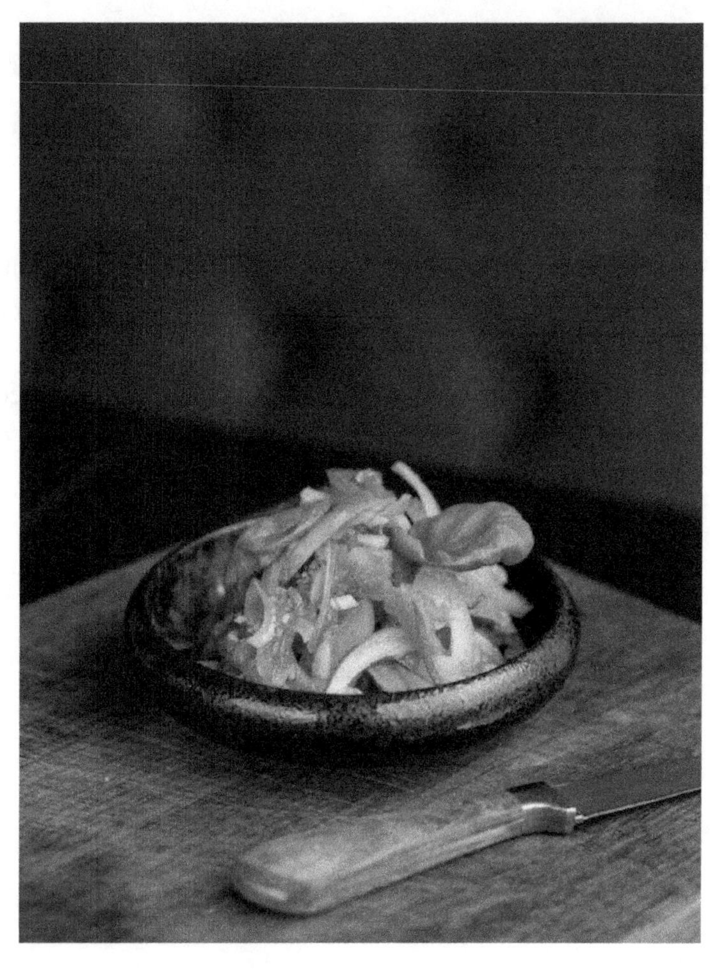

CHAPTER FIVE

Anti-Parkinson's Disease Diet Snack Recipes

1. Nut Butter and Apple Slices

Ingredients:

- Apple, sliced

- Nut butter (almond, peanut, or cashew)

Instructions:

1. Slice an apple into thin rounds.
2. Spread a layer of nut butter on each apple slice.
3. Arrange the slices on a plate and enjoy this simple and nutrient-rich snack.

Preparation Time: 5 minutes

2. Veggie Sticks with Hummus

Ingredients:

- Assorted vegetable sticks (carrots, cucumber, bell peppers, celery)

- Hummus

Instructions:

1. Wash and cut vegetables into sticks.
2. Serve with a side of hummus for dipping.
3. Indulge in this fiber-rich snack that provides vitamins and minerals.

Preparation Time: 10 minutes

3. Trail Mix with Nuts and Berries

Ingredients:

- Mixed nuts (almonds, walnuts, cashews)
- Dried berries (cranberries, blueberries, cherries)
- Dark chocolate chips (optional)

Instructions:

1. Mix together a variety of nuts and dried berries.
2. If desired, add a handful of dark chocolate chips for a touch of sweetness.
3. Portion the trail mix into small containers for convenient snacking.

Preparation Time: 5 minutes

4. Greek Yogurt with Berries and Nuts

Ingredients:

- Greek yogurt

- Mixed berries (blueberries, raspberries, strawberries)

- Chopped nuts (almonds, walnuts)

Instructions:

1. Spoon Greek yogurt into a bowl.

2. Top with a handful of mixed berries and chopped nuts.

3. This protein-packed snack is rich in antioxidants and healthy fats.

Preparation Time: 5 minutes

5. Rice Cakes with Avocado and Tomato

Ingredients:

- Rice cakes

- Avocado, mashed

- Tomato, sliced

- Salt and pepper

- Red pepper flakes (optional, for a kick)

Instructions:

1. Spread mashed avocado on rice cakes.
2. Top with sliced tomato and season with salt, pepper, and red pepper flakes if desired.
3. Savor this crunchy and nutrient-rich snack.

Preparation Time: 5 minutes

Anti Parkinson Disease Diet Smoothies and Juicing Recipes

1. Berry-Banana Brain Boost Smoothie

Ingredients:

- 1 cup mixed berries (blueberries, strawberries, raspberries)
- 1 banana
- 1 cup spinach leaves
- 1 tablespoon chia seeds
- 1/2 cup almond milk (or preferred milk)
- Ice cubes

Instructions:

1. In a blender, combine mixed berries, banana, spinach, chia seeds, almond milk, and ice cubes.
2. Blend until smooth and creamy.
3. Pour into a glass and enjoy this antioxidant-packed smoothie.

Preparation Time: 5 minutes

2. Green Energy Juice

Ingredients:

- 2 green apples, cored and sliced
- 2 celery stalks
- 1 cucumber
- 1 lemon, peeled
- 1-inch piece of ginger

Instructions:

1. Run all the ingredients through a juicer.
2. Stir the juice and pour it into a glass.
3. This refreshing and nutrient-rich green juice can be enjoyed immediately.

Preparation Time: 10 minutes

3. Tropical Turmeric Smoothie

Ingredients:

-   1 cup pineapple chunks

-   1/2 banana

-   1/2 cup mango chunks

-   1 teaspoon turmeric powder

-   1/2 teaspoon ginger, grated

-   1 cup coconut water

-   Ice cubes

Instructions:

1. In a blender, combine pineapple, banana, mango, turmeric, ginger, coconut water, and ice cubes.
2. Blend until smooth and creamy.
3. Pour into a glass and relish this anti-inflammatory and tropical-flavored smoothie.

Preparation Time: 5 minutes

4. Carrot-Orange Immunity Juice

Ingredients:

- 4 large carrots, washed and trimmed
- 2 oranges, peeled and segmented
- 1-inch piece of turmeric root (or 1/2 teaspoon turmeric powder)

Instructions:

1. Run carrots, oranges, and turmeric root through a juicer.
2. Stir the juice and pour it into a glass.
3. This immune-boosting juice is packed with vitamins and antioxidants.

Preparation Time: 10 minutes

5. Creamy Almond Butter Smoothie

Ingredients:

- 1 banana
- 2 tablespoons almond butter
- 1 cup almond milk (or preferred milk)
- 1 tablespoon ground flaxseeds
- 1 teaspoon honey (optional, for sweetness)

-   Ice cubes

Instructions:

1. In a blender, blend banana, almond butter, almond milk, ground flaxseeds, honey, and ice cubes until smooth.
2. Pour into a glass and enjoy this creamy and protein-rich smoothie.

Preparation Time: 5 minutes

CONCLUSION

In conclusion, the role of diet in managing Parkinson's disease cannot be overstated. The concept of an anti-Parkinson's diet emphasizes the significance of specific nutrients, antioxidants, and anti-inflammatory compounds in supporting brain health, managing symptoms, and potentially slowing down the progression of the disease.

While it's important to note that there is no single dietary approach that can cure Parkinson's disease, adopting a well-balanced and nutrient-rich diet can contribute significantly to enhancing the quality of life for individuals living with this condition.

The key components of an anti-Parkinson's diet focus on incorporating foods that are rich in antioxidants, omega-3 fatty acids, lean proteins, whole grains, vitamins, and minerals.

These components collectively work to combat oxidative stress, inflammation, and the loss of dopamine-producing neurons that are characteristic of Parkinson's disease.

The antioxidants found in fruits, vegetables, and certain spices play a crucial role in neutralizing harmful free radicals and protecting brain cells from damage. Omega-3 fatty acids, present in fatty fish, flaxseeds, and walnuts, have anti-inflammatory properties that can help mitigate neurodegenerative processes.

Additionally, the strategic consumption of lean proteins, whole grains, and complex carbohydrates helps stabilize energy levels and regulate blood sugar, preventing fluctuations that can exacerbate both motor and non-motor symptoms of Parkinson's disease.

The inclusion of foods rich in vitamins B6, B12, and folate supports nerve function and aids in reducing homocysteine levels, which have been associated with neurodegeneration.

Furthermore, emerging research highlights the intricate connection between gut health and Parkinson's disease. An anti-Parkinson's diet that includes fiber-rich foods and probiotics supports a healthy gut microbiome, which may have a positive impact on both motor and non-motor symptoms.

9 798858 566519